OASIS

REFRESHING IN NEEDY TIMES

Temitope Ogunsakin BPharm, MSc, PhD

WORDKRAFTIQ

Copyright © 2021 by Temitope Ogunsakin

All rights reserved.

No portion of this book may be reproduced in any form without written permission from the publisher or author, except as permitted by U.S. copyright law.

Contents

Title Page	V
INTRODUCTION	1
PREFACE	6
EPIGRAPH: Desiderata	14
AFTERWORD	16
1. THE BIG PICTURE	19
2. THE BREATH OF LIFE	29
3. THE PRECIOUS MIND	40
4. The Duality of Mind	53
5. THE FOCUSED MIND	62
6. THE HEALING MIND	72
7. MIND CLEANSING	79

8. MINDSET	87
9. GOALS	96
10. CREATIVE VISUALIZATION	105
11. CARING	114
12. TOOLS	123
13. FINAL WORDS	130
14. WORKBOOK	137
15. RESOURCES	140

OASIS

REFRESHING IN NEEDY TIMES

Temitope Ogunsakin BPharm, MSc, PhD

WORDKRAFTIQ

INTRODUCTION

To everything, there ia a season and to every purpose under Heaven. [Eccles. 3:1]

I love to read books; it has been my passion ever since I was a kid; so I lose myself in that world whenever I get the chance. It is therefore no surprise that I do remember almost every book I read while growing up and learning to read! I have spent more time studying various books than in reading for leisure, and a lot more of my money has been spent on books and informative magazines than I have spent on clothing. I have been called a bookworm by those who know me well.

That being said, I respect and am impressed with the diligent work that goes into publishing a book. With this consummate passion therefore, does it surprise anyone that I love to write? I love writing because it makes my day as it fills it with a sense of purpose. And from the poems I scribble on scraps of paper, to the Doodles of on-the -spur-of-the-moment inspiration, major works like OASIS take years of honing and editing. All these writing projects are a form of creativity, and they all of them make my day, every day.

OASIS is a book about the resources within the human mind as provided by Almighty God, the Creator of all. These resources are massively enabling and can be used to awesome benefit for the man or woman who needs to obtain peace and the healing which comes with it. Within the finite time-bound understanding allowed by God and from my humble view, I will take you on a voyage of discovery. It is my sincere hope that this material will meet you at the point of your individual needs as you continue with your journey on life's road.

Everyone's path in life is destiny-specific, with no two destinies being the same, so we will part ways as we choose specific steps that take us to alternate destinations. In OASIS all I have done is to relay my experience while I give practical tips based on my understanding of some issues in life. I hope and pray that this will help you overcome some of the general obstacles which can complicate the stresses in life. These obstacles can always be found in the common aridity that flourishes in societal living. Though they may be found by others with a keen perception, they are mostly taken for granted and overlooked in habitual living with its complacency.

This captivating story of the Brain was first revealed to me one month in the year 2021, the year I suffered a brain stroke. It was by the vantage of inspiration that I was enabled to weather the storm of my affliction. You know how a pebble plops into a still pond, and because it disturbed the stillness, ripples begin to extend radially, even as the causative pebble settles to the murky depths below the surface. The pebble of inspiration unfolded its ripples over the months as I recovered from my affliction, and as two emotions ran rampant in my fuzzy mind. I now generalize these emotions as remorse and shame. I was downcast as I could not speak, and neither could I write or type on my laptop. The very core of my passion was afflicted.

Recovering from a stroke is certainly a miracle! From the vantage threshold of having reduced my inspiration to a printed book just before the stroke about two years earlier, as I review this book for republishing, I keep thanking God profusely for His grace and mercy, my healing, and the expertise of my medical care team. One week after Oasis was first published, I was in the Emergency Department of Houston Medical Center in Warner Robins Georgia battling the ravages of an ischemic stroke. Feeling helpless and frustrated for being unable to say the phrase: 'You can't teach an old dog new tricks', the cognitive and speech assessment. The most miraculous thing that kept assuring me over and over again, was that GOD IS ALWAYS ON THE THRONE OF MERCY!

I had pushed myself to complete the writing of OASIS and finished just a week before, and I completed publishing the first draft.

You may develop a discerning perception as we go on this journey of OASIS, and I pray that is the case. But allow me to state that I am not a teacher but a fellow traveler pointing the way ahead....

Dr. Temitope Ogunsakin

WORDKRAFTIQ PUBLICATIONS

PREFACE

The good thing about life is that every experience is an opportunity to learn. Anyone could write a book from personal life experiences, but we are so immersed in the action that we pass up the opportunity to chronicle events, especially the memorable ones. The great thing about such a book would be the stewardship that drove one's passion and the tips they contain. Though our goals are met when we arrive at our missional destinations and are worth celebrating, we should not miss the 'thrill' of absorbing every bump in our individual journeys while learning from every obstacle. The sweat of life's journey is not only justified by the goal-acquisition, but by the thrill and the value we extract form every experience. I guess what I am trying to say is everyone should know that nothing is a waste in this World of hard knocks.

A book is a compendium of experiences in which an author encapsulates an idea which dropped into his or her consciousness in time. An idea drops into a mind and causes a ripple effect which extensively impacts the mind and the minds of others and when expressed in writing or any other communication, the author's burning desire is fulfilled soon as someone picks up the medium experiencing the words of the author through the mind's eye. From that initiating idea within the author's mind a cascade of words emerged, creating a work of literary art which leads to the reader's experience. Sometimes, the reader of the work, whether fiction or non-fiction, finds agreement with the author's interpretation of the originating idea, and there begins a phenomenon which can only be explained by synergy. I do hope my readers will understand the subject matter of OASIS enough to tell others about it and thank you all in anticipation.

As artworks on a gallery wall are open to interpretation and understanding by individual onlookers, so are the painstaking works of any literary artist. I am honored to be among these inspired men and women. Even though I am no Picasso or Wordsworth, I am passionate about my industry, and am happy you have picked up this copy of OASIS. I pray you will find comfort, thriving peace and wisdom within its pages.

Mindfulness as a practice, helps the Brain create significant mileposts in neuronal pathways and they enable faster and more effective memory recall. Among the other benefits of practicing mindfulness, it can help relieve stress, treat heart disease, lower blood pressure, reduce chronic pain, , improve sleep, and alleviate gastrointestinal difficulties.

But I want to address its effect on memory first. A detailed review of current research suggests that mindfulness helps prevent cognitive decline. Also, mindfulness research shows beneficial effects on attention, processing, and executive functioning. And new research into areas of emotional stress is going on in many countries of the world. Many of us go through our daily lives with a conscious unconsciousness, not fully aware of our conscious experiences. In a discussion moderated by Steve Paulson, executive producer, and host of To the Best of our Knowledge, neuroscientists Richard Davidson and Amishi Jha and clinical mindfulness expert Jon Kabat-Zinn discussed the role of consciousness in mental and physical health on a talk show in 2013. They mentioned how we can train our minds to be more flexible and adaptable, using cutting-edge neuroscience findings about the transformation of consciousness through mindfulness and contemplative practice.

I encourage you to plan to practice a mindful lifestyle for the next 30 days at 5 to 8 minutes a day. You will need to find a comfortable space devoid of distractions while being consistent with the practice.

First, let us get to know the Brain.

I am not a Neurosurgeon, but I have seen impressive Research results even factual and practical truths emerging from the neuro-scientific discoveries of the past 20 years to accentuate the practice of allopathic Medicine and the emerging Wellness paradigm; this emergent paradigm has been the practical use of neuroplasticity to fashion new approaches to brain healing. Very impressive discoveries proving that we can direct our thinking in healthy ways and gain beneficial results.

Every morning as we wake up, new nerve cells are present, which were generated as we slept. Furthermore, work done with neurotransmitters, the basis of brain signals, shows that we can overcome and control depression and anxiety. OASIS has been curated on these premises and much more to give you a good understanding of how you can help leverage neuroplasticity. But what is the fundamental nature of the Brain, expressed in simple terms? To help lay out the information, here are some Brain facts:

The average brain weighs 3Ibs., it is made up of 75% water, generates 23 Watts of electricity, and consumes 20 % of the Body's oxygen.

Many Philosophers, such as Max Ehrmann, the published works of scientists such as Albert Einstein, and the enriching research of such as Jon Kabat-Zinn, speak clearly about the application of mind science. Oasis has been able to digest essential truths and use the result to lead you to an oasis of rejuvenation and restoration.

Since this book is about finding daily solace in which the Oasis of the brain can provide the required renewal that it is wired to facilitate, I have taken the liberty to quote one of my favorite writings. The article is written by Max Ehrmann and titled "Desiderata" (Latin: "things desired"). It is an early 1920s piece by this American writer. I had held it dear since my College days when things were very rough, and I needed comfort and restoration. It was given to me on a torn piece of paper by a friend I thought did not know what he had just handed me. Why? Because I was assisting him in moving to a new house, and it was in a pile of trash.

I have always valued the feel of paper and the contents of paper which may prove valuable. I learned this when I avidly collected stamps, staring at the minor works of philatelic art and the information they bore from other places around the globe. So, on that fateful Saturday morning, I was helping Don to clear his room preparatory to moving. He gave me a pile of magazines and odd papers; right in the middle of one time-aged magazine was the poem by Max Ehrmann. I did not discover it till I returned to my College apartment, all worn out after so much heavy lifting. With a few bucks in hard-earned wages for my pain, I flopped into the armchair in my one-room apartment. I propped up my feet and went through what I subconsciously felt was the most valuable outcome of my chores for that day. (I told you I have a bond with paper). I went through the pile of magazines Don had bequeathed me, and it was about the third in the pile that I made a unique discovery. Having tossed the previous two magazines into 'true' trash, I was flipping through the pages browned with time and dust, and there it was! Third, in a pile, I came across a piece of paper frayed at the edges. Across its top, I read the words: 'Desiderata,' which I must confess I knew nothing about its meaning at the time. As we explore the literary World, we find that some people have been given a mastership of words and have also been crowned with the inspiration to deliver those words with appropriateness that lives beyond time. Such a man was Max Ehrmann; his work is a great inspiration, and Desiderata is an enabler worth quoting in OASIS.

Indeed, Mr. Ehrmann alludes to the Oasis's existence and the efficacy of the waters from its deep wells to revitalize and rejuvenate those who are thirsty and exhausted from Life's afflictions. I invite you to read this copy of Desiderata.

('Desiderata' means things that are desired or wanted. The implication is that these are desired qualities of the soul and heart.)

EPIGRAPH: Desiderata

Go placidly amid the noise and the haste; remember what peace there may be in silence. As far as possible, without surrender, be on good terms with all persons. Speak your truth quietly and clearly, and listen to others, even to the dull and the ignorant; they, too, have their story.

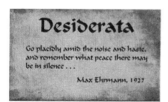

Avoid loud and aggressive people. They are vexatious to the spirit. If you compare yourself with others, you may become vain or bitter, for always there will be greater and lesser persons than yourself. Enjoy your achievements as well as your plans. Keep interested in your career, however humble; it is a real possession in the changing fortunes of time. Exercise caution in your business affairs, for the World is full of trickery. But let this not blind you to what virtue there is; many persons strive for high ideals, and everywhere Life is full of heroism. Be yourself. Especially do not feign affection. Neither be cynical about love, for, in the face of all aridity and disenchantment, it is as perennial as the grass. Take kindly the counsel of the years, gracefully surrendering the things of youth. Nurture strength of spirit to shield you in sudden misfortune. But do not distress yourself with dark imaginings. Many fears are born of fatigue and loneliness. Beyond a wholesome discipline, be gentle with yourself. You are a child of the universe no less than the trees and the stars: you have a right to be here. And whether it is clear to you, no doubt the universe is unfolding as it should. Therefore, be at peace with God, whatever you conceive Him to be. And whatever your labors and aspirations, in the noisy confusion of Life, keep peace in your soul. With all its sham, drudgery, and broken dreams, it is still a beautiful world. Be cheerful. Strive to be happy.   [Desiderata was written by Max Ehrmann in 1927]

AFTERWORD

It was once believed that when damage to the Brain occurred, there was little hope of recovery. We now know that this is not true. The brain is constantly changing, in an effort to function the best that it can; and, crucially, to heal itself after damage.

As a Pharmacist practicing for many years before my stroke, I didn't know as much about the Brain as I do now. I am trying to tell my readers that prevention, recovery, and survival are equally important in preserving Brain health.

The Brain is an amazingly complex organ that manages everything we think, feel, and do. When an individual suffers a stroke such as I did, the poor blood flow to the brain causes cell-death and a cascade of physiological dyscrasias. Pathways of communication from one area of the brain to another are disrupted. The textbooks speak of two main types of stroke: ischemic, due to lack of blood flow, and hemorrhagic, which is due to bleeding which causes parts of the brain to stop functioning properly.

Oasis is from the pen of a Stroke Survivor. Three-quarters of the initial script had been completed about one week before the stroke happened. All through the trauma and hospitalization my world was a vague whirl of despondency. But one month later I had bounced back on the road to full recovery. From the anguish of speech disability, right-arm non-functionality, and the throes of Aphasia, Almighty God healed me to tell my story. I will praise God for I am fearfully and wonderfully made. [Psalm 139:14]

OASIS is the refreshing everyone needs for a proactive plan in the prevention of the neuro-fatigue of a stress-filled existence. It contains valid and practical information for all, and it gets better with application.

Every Survivor has an opportunity to be restored in health and functionality, but at the end of it all, survivors must prevent future reoccurrences as much as possible. Since the terrain is different for everyone and experiences differ, we all have to virtually work with whatever circumstance our environment provides. Oasis will grant you the rest and healing you required.

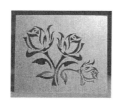

Chapter 1

THE BIG PICTURE

More to see

There is more to see than meets the eye! It is a big wide world which, though we cannot grasp the extent and vastness of it, we can do occasional snapshots in the realization that the Creator is a Master at the Art of micronizing the Universe, even in a grain of sand. We can learn a lot from our immediate circumstance. One thing that is clear is that the human mind operates as an instrument of immense capacity and awesome depth. According to a recent article in Scientific American, the memory capacity of the human brain was testified to have equal to 2.5 petabytes of memory capacity. A "petabyte" means 1024 terabytes or million gigabytes. Therefore, the brain can accumulate the equivalent of 2.5 million gigabytes of memory, of which it is said that we use only 10%!

We are going to explore some of the depths of reality in OASIS, and I want you to enjoy the ride!

As individuals, we constantly stare at our feet instead of looking at where we are going and occasionally encounter obstacles. Obstacles are not really negative in the final analysis when we consider that we can always emerge stronger and wiser after we have surmounted the obstacle. Not always having eyes on our goals, we tend to be more reactive than proactive, whereas proactivity is an enabling state of anticipation and readiness. Proactive mindfulness is the best antidote for debilitating surprises (this is another phrase for accidents). After reading this book, you will apply a new style with a more current and cogent approach to your reality. Your reality results from sensory activities and is related to your environment. Your reality is a 'truth,' a law for your existence that impacts your physiology and your

Health & Wellness. Your truth is your mindset because your mind is set on it, but very potent as they affect our moods and emotions. Your truth is your reality, a law that guides your existence and can make things happen for you. Your truth helps to bring things into your environment or blocks you from realizing a thing. Unless you bypass it, it will remain a prime influence. OASIS is not a new invention, but a synergy of many forms that have proven to help many people form practical personal lifestyles. As I developed the OASIS template through continuous improvement, I borrowed from many well-researched methodologies, such as the work and research of Dr. Jon Kabat Zin. I jokingly say but earnestly believe that Almighty God owns the only valid copyright in Life. Even when you borrow from His examples, He does not flood you with litigations for infringement! Published Research stimulates further Research, and only in meta-analysis is the big picture seen. We often do not have a broad view because we sit in the big picture afflicted by a short sightedness. For example, I started using a 'tool' in my Primary School days, having stumbled across it unknowingly. I had struggled in the lower ranks of the Class, but when I discovered this rudimentary method, it seemed as if a window which had been draped with black curtains had those curtains ripped away. The previous stygian darkness seemingly disappeared. Within weeks, I was at the top of my Class and remained there till I graduated and went to College. And even now that I am retired, I still use the tool after many years of practicing Pharmacy. I have seen a fragment of the commercially available mind-maps tool, but my tool has much more in it than is commercially available. By the time we end our trip into OASIS, you will have started to assemble your own tool for personal effectiveness. I am helping you create a passion that is the core element of personal effectiveness. Observing the world of personal growth tools, I see a need for a tool like the one presented in OASIS.

Feeling stuck or powerless in Life happens often, but it is only through the grace of a receding memory that we walk with hope and strength and tackle this life of hard knocks and we are not bogged down by a remorseful memory for long. This sounds like an oxymoron. A receding memory as time passes is a safety-mechanism since some memories can be traumatic. These memories sometimes generate a fear of an unknown result, to the extent that it kills the urge to try again whatever brought failure in the past. Also, this fading could serve as 'red flags' which can spur a discerning mind to remember to exercise the brain. For when the memory starts to get fuzzy, it may be time to recharge the brain. There will be more examples of how to recharge the brain within this book.

Sometimes, the words people speak, and our own self-speak can trigger a cascade of neurochemicals within our physiology and the main parts of the brain. The brain's self-cleansing mechanism protects us from an overload of anxiety in present circumstances, provided we can escape a mindset of interference which would degrade this effective and natural maintenance process. Despite what may come to mind, getting out of this interfering mindset is an act which yields results, and not one which tries to force results. The brain has a self-cleansing mechanism that tries to protect us from an overload of the effects of anxiety and stress in present circumstances. This protection is quite effective provided we can escape the habitual mindset of overriding Nature's beneficial suggestions.

MIND POTENTIAL

The tool I mentioned will help you develop a methodology for greater personal productivity, good results-orientation, and being vibrant while opening your understanding to a beneficial principle. This fundamental principle is the Law of Potential. This Law of Potential (distilled from Science and observed phenomena) operates whether one recognizes it or not. The Law stands outside the door of reality and is ready to unfold once anyone opens the door to opportunity. Though, the door does not open by itself, it is no respecter of persons. The door of opportunity will allow its choice to be molded, directed, or stopped by the human mind since the mind's wish is its command. Using this key to open the door of abundance means knowing that this door exists. Yes! The potential is abundant in you. You will realize your true potential and activate it if you do not give up. I wish to appeal to that subconscious drive within you that says, 'Why not?' If others who went before can, why not you? Dare to try! When you succeed, it will be because you decided to take a meaningful step, the vital step. The answer to this question is vital to completing any successful journey. Since to be successful, one must equip oneself appropriately and prevent taking any wrong turns or using unnecessary diversions on the road ahead. Let us look at some specifics. Each 24-hour day is full of precious NOW ZONES. A Now Zone is an enabling moment in time when the Genius in everyone is optimally primed for potential effectiveness. This knowledge is the key to abundance, for there are many gateways of revelation represented by what I call a NOW ZONE each day. All you need is one inspirational moment for critical and enabling momentum. Go through the gateway provided by the Now Zone, and on the other side lies a potential 'aha' moment. It could be the memory fragment you have endlessly searched for. A search like this could possibly go on for months with no results to show. Or maybe this search was for the vital lynchpin to a groundbreaking design; a search which may have proven elusive till now. So, be at peace with yourself and reflect on every one of life's graces. You will be astounded by the treasures you will discover.

When you are at peace, your anxiety is diverted but not destroyed, since energy cannot be destroyed. The diversion of your anxiety essentially frees your brain's resources while allowing it to be constructive. Therefore, contemplate the little things that may have been taken for granted prior to now. Be grateful knowing that you were blessed with them for a purpose. This little exercise will yield great rewards. Also, observe the Sunrise each morning, and if you are privileged to see the birds make their morning rounds as they sing on the wing or twig. Try to observe as they trust and love Nature for her immense generosity.

Every chapter of OASIS will end with an applicative tool which I have named the synoptic applicative tool (SAT). SAT will further help the reader to recollect essential key points in the chapter allowing us to link them in a strategy for moving forward as we attain our set goals.

APPLICATION: YOU ARE HERE AND NOW

Your mind has a large expanse of undeveloped potential which can further be developed and improved upon in the NOW ZONE. We all are meant to give more to the World, and I am convinced that every life experience is an extra layer of learning, that over time, will prepare us to effectively interact with life's circumstances. Along the way, every pain experienced is a birthing and a catharsis, and every disappointment is a door that didn't open to a distraction. Whatever is your experience, you should learn that life is one lifelong vital lesson in patience. Indeed, every lesson in patience is meant to accentuate a positive virtue and provide a test leading to endurance. So, my dear friend, persevere as you must, and while enduring the many tests, remember that the finest steel requires lots of heat and intermittent cooling in-between the hot spots. For you, the cooling period is when you come out of the proverbial desert and apply a method that you will learn from this book: OASIS.

I wish you all the best for thriving and I anticipate your good success.

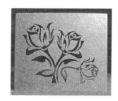

THE BREATH OF LIFE

Be mindfuol of your thriving

The Human Brain is an arena of storms, but in the midst of it all, can be found creativity and healing. In life we are on a constant treadmill, a mixed terrain of reality, from sunrise to the setting of the same Sun. A treadmill is the term I use to describe the endless repetition of stress-related routines in everyday living which do not produce any results of value. Our reality defines our circumstances in life and since we are given custody of this reality through our senses, we can mold our circumstances to a large degree if we want to.

While recognizing that lifestyle choices form a substantial part of the complexity of life, I have used my research in adult learning and motivation coupled with the latest neuroscientific publications and mindfulness findings, to craft the OASIS method.

To appease the savage beast of modern-day living, we must get off this perpetual treadmill as safely and quickly as possible, so we can apply the tool of mindfulness. Indeed, there are many upsides to adopting a focused mindful lifestyle. This is why I also recommend the process is mentioned in SYN-O-VATE, a toolkit for would-be Entrepreneurs. Some of the benefits of Syn-o-vate are:

Discovering that you have potential you never knew you had, finding pockets of time you thought you never had , and an improved Health and Wellness. As you go about your tasks with more vigor and effectiveness, there will be an enabling factor which predisposes your efforts to further success.

A simple summary of OASIS is a simple statement:

THRIVING IN LIFE THROUGH APPLIED MINDFULNESS.

Thriving allows you to feel better, having better health, and an excellent holistic balance. There is a more vibrant outlook on life which is crucial for us to attain the emotional balance required for a healthy and prosperous life. Remember, illness or feeling unwell is the body's way of letting you know that something is out of balance. This feeling leads to procrastination, brain fog, and a lack of drive. Being subdued by a lack of drive is a common affliction in today's World, and it tends to defeat both the young and not-so-young in their aspirations.

In OASIS, the practice of consistent mindfulness helps to maximize your internal resources making you more effective as a person. For example, supposing you are not 'listening' to what your body is saying, you will miss that inaudible but consistent 'voice.' A voice that has guided many through the ages. It pays to learn the language of this vital resource, learning that can be accumulated daily. In a consistent five-minute a-day practice, you will get clear of the confusion that is stress.

These results are obtained in the Now Zone, where we hear what the mind's intimate voice says to those who listen.

To listen to what the mind is saying, one must get off the treadmill of a humdrum life for at least five minutes daily. Regular doses of these five-minute sessions will lead to a cascading effect, and I want you to try it with great anticipation. Well, here is the rationale behind that:

As you accumulate your experiences in the Now Zone, something becomes noticeable:

On close observation, you will notice, over time, that you have become a more effective time economist. Becoming a more effective time economist means being more proactive in crucial activities and, therefore becoming more result-oriented in applying your skills. I am now an eternal student of this methodology, since I became convinced that 'time' as a wasting resource, is vital to effective stewardship of all Nature has blessed us with.

Since everyone's consciousness is time-bound and consciousness rules our reality, it follows that existence and life's activities, is based on a time-measured consciousness. If we can use time effectively, we can better interact with our reality and walk the paths of life using mind resources efficiently .

The gateway of reality is the small window in the hourglass of my consciousness; the Now. Mindful meditation in the Now helps calm stress hormones, and nothing beats an excellent proactive stress-management system. The adverse effects of stress are best prevented than healed. OASIS is a vital resource that gives you a winning game plan.

Finally, I must say this, so it does not get lost in the sandy paths of our journey to the Oasis, while reading this book. Central to the bunch of techniques that we have called OASIS is BREATH. Of equal importance is the MIND but let us remember that BREATH gives Life without which the mind would not be active. So, let us spend some time exploring this source of our vitality. Since we are blessed with an innate ability to breathe unconsciously, it is not surprising that breath is rarely considered in the Healing Arts, except in the Eastern philosophies.

In India, there is a Sanskrit proverb that says:

Breath is life; if you breathe well, you will live long on Earth.

Breathing pervades all cultures of the World and all the classifications which unite or separate the Human Race. Everybody is breathing! It even influences other divisions of flora and fauna in Nature. It is the essential factor necessary to sustain Life. From the first breath at birth to the last one taken just before transitioning into the next Life, everyone will take approximately half a billion breaths in one lifetime. Consciously or unconsciously, human breath is influenced by our thoughts, so learning to apply consciousness to our breathing pattern is a valuable tool in helping us restore essential balance to mind and body. When chosen as a lifetime strategy, mindfulness helps the practitioner leverage innate strengths that an individual may be unaware of possessing. Due to its de-stressing potency, mindfulness meditation helps eliminate acidic toxins from the body. You will find OASIS links deep breathing, mindfulness meditation, and wellness through these applications. OASIS is a synergistic synthesis of mindfulness practice, researched facts & data, and Health & Wellness. Coming from the proven premise that the Human mind is central to physiological, psychological, and spiritual functions.

A lack of drive is a common affliction in today's World that tends to defeat both the young and not-so-young in their aspirations. With OASIS, your internal resources will become more effective, and effectiveness goes together with tracking and measuring your continuous performance. For example, let us suppose you are not 'listening to what the body is saying. In that case, you will miss it since it is an inaudible though consistent 'voice.' The fourth item in the concise list of results (page 23) to expect as you disembark the treadmill says that your resources will

These results are obtained in the Now Zone, where we hear what the mind's intimate voice says to those who listen.

To understand what the mind is saying, one must get off the treadmill of a humdrum life for at least 10 minutes daily. Regular doses of these 10-minute sessions will lead to a cascading effect, and I want you to try it when you expect a miracle. Well, here is the rationale behind that:

As you accumulate your experiences in the Now Zone, something becomes noticeable:

On close observation, you will notice, over time, that you have become a more effective time economist. Becoming a more effective time economist means being more proactive in crucial activities and, therefore, more result-oriented in applying definite skills. I am now an eternal student of this methodology since I became convinced that 'time' as a wasting resource, is vital to effective stewardship of all Nature has blessed us with,

Since everyone's consciousness is time-bound and consciousness rules our reality, it follows that existence or whatever is fundamental to us is based on a time-measured consciousness. If we can use time effectively, we can better interact with our reality and walk the paths of prosperity.

The gateway of reality is the small window in the hourglass of my consciousness; the Now. Mindful meditation in the Now helps calm stress hormones, and nothing beats an excellent proactive stress-management system. The adverse effects of stress are best prevented than healed. OASIS is a vital resource that gives you a winning game plan.

Finally, I must say this for fear that it may get lost as we step through the sandy paths in our journey to the Oasis while reading this book. Central to the bunch of techniques that we have called OASIS is BREATH. Of equal importance is the MIND but let us remember that BREATH gives Life without which the mind would not be active. So, let us spend some time exploring this vital resource, which, unfortunately, is taken for granted. Since we are blessed with an innate ability to breathe unconsciously, it is unsurprising that breath is rarely considered in the Healing Arts.

In India, there is a Sanskrit proverb that says:

Breath is life; if you breathe well, you will live long on Earth.

Breathing pervades all cultures of the World and all the classifications which unite or separate the Human Race. Everybody is breathing! It even influences other divisions of flora and fauna in Nature. It is the essential factor necessary to sustain Life. From the first breath at birth to the last one taken just before transitioning into the next Life, everyone will take approximately half a billion breaths in one lifetime. Consciously or unconsciously, human breath is influenced by our thoughts, so learning to apply consciousness to our breathing pattern is a valuable tool in helping us restore essential balance to mind and body. When chosen as a lifetime strategy, mindfulness helps the practitioner leverage innate strengths that an individual may be unaware of possessing. Due to its de-stressing potency, mindfulness meditation helps eliminate acidic toxins from the body. You will find OASIS links deep breathing, mindfulness meditation, and wellness through these applications. OASIS is a synergistic synthesis of mindfulness practice, researched facts & data, and Health & Wellness. Coming from the proven premise that the Human mind is central to physiological, psychological, and spiritual functions.

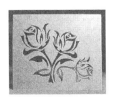

Chapter 3

THE PRECIOUS MIND

A Pristine Diamond

OASIS is a compendium of facts-and-data that leads you gradually to access a productive lifestyle of result-oriented application of mindfulness. The mind-activating process laid out in this book is a method that has helped me overcome the debilities of an ischemic stroke, the health devastation of congestive heart failure, and the depression that sets-in when you feel that life is just slipping by. This book will help to attain a conducive frame of mind in which your spirit is energized as you step into Life with increased vibrancy and deeper understanding. Closely examine your thoughts, and always polish those ones that lead you to higher aspirations. Thoughts have wings, and lofty thoughts have the ability to fly high, propelling you far into the arena of good success in your endeavors. Thoughts are gems ; every snowflake of thought has the potential to become part of the cascading avalanche of success if it gathers momentum. This momentum is what OASIS is all about. And since all our gains on this journey will be traceable to the initial steps we take, no matter in which direction those steps lead, when we ask, 'How did these steps start?' one thing that will be common to every answer will be: 'The initial steps started in mind'.

Dear Reader, I want to share a story with you, titled: Acres of Diamonds. It is a story that has stood the test of time and a classic that generations of young and old folks have read. It has been orally shared beside campfire flames for hundreds of years. This story has led many people to rethink their Life's strategy, and If you have not read it before, I suggest you find a copy and dive into its fascinating depths. You will find an exotic and enriching account of the benefits of patience; the rewards of applying a patient examination to our day-to-day decision-making, for there are rewards to be garnered in every moment of thoughtfulness. Slowing down the frenetic pace dictated by modern society, and being more thoughtful as we make critical decisions, leads one to a winning start.

Written by Russell Conwell, born in Massachusetts in 1843; he served during the Civil War as a Captain in the Union Army. After studying Law, he became a Baptist Minister and a public speaker.

The material in the book was Conwell's famous talk which he delivered on over 6000 crowded occasions. He could be named as one of the original motivational speakers. The story's core is based on a parable that Conwell had heard while traveling in Iraq in 1870. The book has the theme: *opportunity lurks in everyone's backyard*. So true!

ACRES OF DIAMONDS by Russell Conwell

(abridged excerpt follows)

Once, a wealthy man named Ali Hafed had his home near the River Indus. One day a Priest visited Ali Hafed and, in conversation after Dinner, told him a tale about diamonds. Ali Hafed was in amazement, listening to the Priest. The value in such small quantities of gems was almost unimaginable! When Ali went to bed, he had his imagination ablaze. Throughout the dream all he thought about was what he could do with such incredible wealth. So, in the morning, when he awoke, he quickly decided to sell his farm and go on a journey to seek his wealth in Diamonds.

He packed up a few belongings and left on a journey without any further guidance but the story from an old Priest who had heard stories repeated to his hearing from mere hearsay. Ali Hafed believed that he was stepping into a World full of diamonds and riches. He left his old farm in the hands of the new owner, his neighbor, and leaving his family behind, he traveled to Palestine and continued into Europe looking for priceless baubles. After many years of grueling and fruitless search, his health started to fail, and all the money he had received from the sale of his farm had fizzled out. Morose and heartbroken, he threw himself into the sea to kill himself.

One day, thousands of miles away, and at the end of a very extensive weeding run, the neighbor who purchased Ali's farm had decided to call it a day after tending farm all day. So, he went to the nearby stream of water to wash up. As he dipped himself into the cool and sparkling water, he made sure he kept an eye out for snakes, as lately, he had spotted a few. As he repeatedly dipped in the cool waters of the stream, he noticed a scintillating flicker of light. Thinking it was the evening sun playing games with his vision, he dipped slower into the water while keeping his eyes trained on the same spot, getting ready to jump in case he spotted any slithery movement. The flash of light was unmistakable! That was what caught his eye. So, he reached out with hesitant fingers, and indeed he felt a piece of rock wedged in the bed of the stream. He could not believe his eyes as he pulled it out of the water, It was the largest diamond he had ever seen! When he ran into the house with it, his wife Kudirat thought he must have been drinking again. But she saw what he held in his hands; she almost fainted! It is said that this was the beginning of the discovery of the famed Diamonds of Golconda. The Golconda region has produced some of the World's most famous diamonds, including the colorless Koh-i-Noor, now owned by the United Kingdom.

All through the years in which Ali had farmed his stretch of land, it had yielded just a few lean harvests, but unknown to him that farm had always sat on top of an extraordinarily rich and extensive Diamond field. One significant benefit I derived from this story is that careful thought, not an impulsive one, is more rewarding than the circumstances rushing at us.

Have you ever received a phone call asking you to drop whatever you were doing and rush across town to an unplanned activity? Have you been called by a friend who engaged you in endless conversation on the phone? Do you wake up in the morning, and for the first hour, you do not know what you will do early in the morning? I could go on all day with a list of scenarios where all of us, one way or the other, get precious moments 'stolen' from us without knowing we have lost a gem waiting to be polished. I am here to let you know that a special moment lost can never be regained! Everyone has a moment of genius, at least on any 24-hour day, if only we are not looking elsewhere when it slips by. Through OASIS, you will begin to identify these precious moments. They usually occur as we wake up in the morning, or they could happen when we find time away from a crowd, not being distracted by phone calls or T.V., the 'echoing' silence could grow on you.

But as you learn the art of introspection, you will find diamonds at the introspective moment if you closely examine the thoughts that pop up. In crafting your style, and it is a personal one, you will need to nail down your first objective, which is:

Plan to spend 10 minutes of now-mindfulness every day (better if it is the first thing you do in the morning). Even if you have another 10-minute session later in the day, you would have opened the window to the genius-flow first thing that morning. A passionate practice of this 10-minute strategy unlocks the genius. Passion is the genesis of genius.

LIFE'S OBJECTIVE

Everyone's life's objective is colored by continuous glimpses of a vision and an understanding of purpose. Being that life's purpose is never given in a blueprint, you will understand why I used the phrase: 'continuous glimpses'. A gradual discovery of the compass of purpose is usually made in the traveler's bag while digging for one thing or another, apparently neatly tucked away by the same Hand that fashioned destiny. The purpose of one's existence is a necessary discovery in any lifetime, it is what gives the expanse of years its color; it qualifies every objective while giving it the necessary meaning. Without purpose, we would be gambling life away in the school of hard knocks. As I write this book, though the vision was known, the purpose was not spelled out at the beginning. It emerged and got clearer as the chapters evolved; with a cascade of words, the ship of 'OASIS' has brought me to remote shores and distant lands, emerging in color and forms which beat my imagination. For me, it has been an awe-inspiring self-discovery, and I hope it will transform your life.

Set your vision for the long run about your goals and for what lies in-between as well! Goals are the mileposts we must attain on our way to our established visions, so every day, one must review goals in a way that allows us to understand the progress that is made toward each identified vision or objective. Please remember that living in the moment will allow us to identify other critical inputs for the journey which lies ahead. Understanding the elements essential for key moments will equip each one of us with a proactive ability to succeed even when faced with unknown odds. Everyone is helped when we find momentary opportunities in the transient but daily opening of the window of genius. The time of opening is not declared but makes the opportunity worth our while. In History, from Archimedes to the Wright Brothers and from Thomas Edison to John Washington Carver, we see individuals utilizing the window of genius. John Washington Carver learned to tap into the momentary and incredible power of the NOW. In the NOW, those with access can witness the rewarding experience of the opening widow of genius.

Some, in History have succeeded in opening the path to their daily inspiration, which is represented by the term 'window of genius'. According to J.W. Carver, he said:

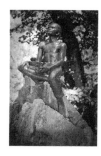
"No books ever go into my laboratory. The thing I am to do is revealed to me the moment I am inspired to create something new. Without God to draw aside the curtain, I would be helpless. Only alone can I draw close enough to God to discover His secrets." John Washington Carver

GETTING THINGS DONE

Goals: Mileposts on the way to your Vision.

The mind is a mirror of the Soul. It is a reflective and collective vessel for the Creator's abundance. It is a pristine lake in the gentle breeze which reflects the glory of God upon life. As above, so below. The Heavens reflects the glory of God!

Outside of you, it could be a raging tornado, but you should always seek the eye-of-the-storm within, which is a Divine peace. A quiet mind gets things done. You may not be able to change the elements and the way the World behaves, but you can change yourself through your perception and, by the same process, your reality.

Within the pages of OASIS, there are multiple mentions of SYN-O-VATE a resource I have published to encourage entrepreneurs in all of us. It serves to help keep the momentum going.

WHAT IS SYN-O-VATE?

Synovate is a coaching tool for energizing breakthroughs and is very useful for enhancing effectiveness especially when the individual's effort requires self-motivation, drive, and diligence. Synovate is a useful tool to have in every entrepreneurial tool bag. It brings together aspects of your inner genius to explore innovative ways of getting things done.

More details will be made available on the website http://www.temgun.com

APPLICATION: A PRODUCTIVE OBJECTIVE

Your true life's objective is a precious diamond that resides in your mind, preserve and nurture it.

You will get things done better with a quietened mind.

Without understanding life's objective, one would wander the paths of life aimlessly. The man who finds meaning in life is one who comes alive with a passion to live while enjoying the true meaning of the journey, and to find the truth for one's life is to understand its object.

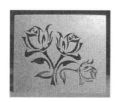

Chapter 4

The Duality of Mind

Reclaim vital assetts

The Human Mind is a Quarterback in the game of life. As a Quarterback directs the game on the field of play in American football, so it is with the mind. It is an existential conscious entity that directs the assemblage of processes that contribute to life and consciousness. The mind's playbook is hidden in what we know as the recesses of memory, with complex play- styles and self-adjusting tactics. How and when these tactics are deployed depends on intricate sensory signals mediated by the brain and various arrays of nerves, chemicals, and substrates. Everyone knows that in the game of football, all the players should possess good physical and technical prowess as well as quickly responsive learning skills. All these qualities can be ascribed to the Human Mind. The Human Mind is a composite. A composite which allows us to go about many activities while not being distracted. One half of the composite is called the conscious mind, and the other half is called the subconscious mind. An important aspect of our work with the strategies of the Human mind mindfulness as it opens the door into the playbook as described. As one hopes to catch a wild bird with open hands, we virtually have to proceed with stealth and wisdom. The truth is that the mind empowers itself by storing its unused elements in the depths of memory. When we lose track of a thing or cannot remember things we had experienced in the past, our attempts to recall are like trying to squeeze juice from a hard green lemon. It is almost futile in every attempt to consciously retrieve forgotten memories; so, we need to adopt a new approach. Just as the green lemon ripens without any conscious intervention, we need to use a more subtle technique. The Chinese idiom says: Softly, softly catchee monkey. This technique is applied in the now zone. Paying mindful attention to our breath, we avoid all distraction from the quietness and allow the sensation of breath to balance our higher senses. In this zone of mindfulness, the brain synapses are allowed to 'breathe' and refresh. A refreshed brain usually opens up to exploration. The flood of neurotransmitters that is usually generated in stress, and which transferring nerve impulses, lead to a form of overthinking; thus slowing neuronal communication. This is a type of brain fog making us less productive, demotivated and less focused. The Paying-mindful attention to breath exercise, the reversal takes place, and the brain gets refreshed. This is why I recommend SYN-O-VATE. Those of us who do a lot of thinking about issues and stress a lot, need to try this.

The Chinese base their impressive Philosophy on the concept of Duality, and it is called Yin and Yang. Typifying every occurrence by this harmonious 'opposition', they identify some as Male and others in the opposite, as Female. There are two sides toa coin; every day starts with sunrise and ends with sunset. For everything that the mind conceives, it can easily come up with an opposite thought, object, or dream. We know that you cannot have black without white, and you cannot have empty without full. Contemplating the opposites in Duality is a good war-up for starting a mindfulness discipline. These dualities speak to the fundamental truth of what gives Life meaning and power. it is the Duality that starts the 'coloring process' of our various circumstances in Life. Eventually, this coloring process tones our emotions and our aspirations, and if not well understood, will cause us to 'walk' in pathways that do not conform to our real plans and destination.

The Greeks got it partially right. Their philosophy was binary in nature. Male and Female, good and evil, light and dark, and so on. The problem is that the Greeks focused primarily on the 'good things', the ideals, the forms, and the essence. When they did this, they side-lined the other half of the equation. What does the Holy Bible say in this matter?

My favorite reference scriptures are to be found in Genesis and Ecclesiastes:

Genesis 1:1 speaks of a beginning.

"In the beginning, God created the heaven and the Earth."

In this portion of scripture, the beginning of the Holy text, there is an indication of the Duality which was the start of the whole Creation story. And in the book of Ecclesiastes, we are introduced to one of the rudimentary representations of Duality in time. From being born and dying, planting, and harvesting, killing, and healing, breaking down and building; Ecclesiastes 3:1-8 speaks about a series of events: from being born and dying, planting, and harvesting, killing, and healing, breaking down and building up, weeping, and laughing, mourning, and dancing, throwing stones and gathering stones, embracing, and not embracing, acquiring things and losing things, keeping together and throwing away, tearing apart and sewing up, keeping silence and speaking, loving and hating, making war and seeking peace. Without stretching our imagination extensively, we quickly realize that we live in a World of manifested dualities. We learn through reading Ecclesiastes, that by focusing only on the positives in matter, at the expense of the anti-matter and on light at the expense of darkness, we have stripped away a significant portion of the power of Duality. The Western mind has historically viewed the other side of these equations as suspect or weak or somehow untrustworthy. It is easy to celebrate the masculine side of personality, but we are suspicious of the female side. It is easy to value the light, but we fear the darkness. This is the Greek or Western mindset.

This is an alternative to the Greek black and white mindset.

The 'Yin and the Yang'. When you look at the Yin and Yang symbol, it is obvious that it acknowledges the binary nature of reality. but unlike westerners, the Chinese see an equal value on the other side of the equation.

They understand that "full" or "substance" would be meaningless without the complimentary reality of "emptiness" or "nothingness".

One good example of this is in the Tao Te Ching, the primary scripture of Taoism, where it highlights the importance of the empty hole in a pot. Usually, people do not think about the empty hole. But the Tao Te Ching points out that it is the emptiness inside the pot that gives it its value, after all, that is where you store stuff. A solid pot with no hole in the middle is completely worthless. In other words, it is the void or the nothingness that exists in a binary relationship with something that gives life value. This is how you get a big picture of the eternal. You go past Duality and understand and ultimately embrace the Power of the void.

The idea of Duality communicates this loud and clear. You cannot see, touch, taste, smell, and hear, but it is real, nonetheless. The key which turns on the process of realization, however, is focus. Focus is the driver of human realization. Focus excludes distractions and helps the mind stay in areas where the mind is set on one thing at a time.

RECLAMATION

With OASIS, you are adopting a mindset that uses mindfulness and a disciplined focus to reclaim valuable time which is inadvertently lost through distractions, thus helping you to sustain a steady course in the days ahead. I suggest that you let the lifestyle sink in by aiming to consistently live an OASIS lifestyle for an initial 30-days. By disciplining your powers of observation, you will gain an improved perspective that will unlock many opportunities for innovation. Remember that your chosen moment of mindfulness needs not go on for more than ten minutes. As you flow with your conscious breath, you are not focused on distractive activities or worrisome issues. Your mind will spring free with an abundance of previously wasted potential energy. In your newfound liveliness, creativity and effectiveness become your allies and enablers. Since you are in the presence of self in the here and-now, self will also assist you to apply this immense potential to areas you may not have thought of before. The techniques that you learn in OASIS work with how your mind is already configured. You are not doing something new to your Brain. You are just tapping abilities it already has. It all boils down to shifting your focus and energy. Everything else will flow because the mind already has mechanisms ready to swing into action. However, proceed carefully and write notes. Assume the caution of a young boy learning to ride his new bike.

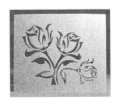

Chapter 5

THE FOCUSED MIND

Parting the veil purposefully

As each day brings its challenges, your focus and inner calm are the two conditions that may help guarantee that you will successfully navigate the day's course: they are important factors in overcoming whatever challenges you may face. You may have multiple College degrees or the best I.Q. in the World. However, the explosiveness of Life's cascade of challenges is best defused from a different perspective. Using the term 'focus' is not the word's common meaning. We do not mean to concentrate. It connotes the opposite. We will focus on the moment and let everything else go. We use the word here to mean 'staying in the zone'

The zone is synonymous with 'the moment'. The zone has no visible boundaries and is not a room or specific location. The zone is the 'now' moment. Its location is in time and it is bound by consciousness. The now is not present when you are asleep or unconscious, being a fragment of perspective in your conscious mind frame. There is a personal zone that belongs to you where you can enable factors that speak to your ultimate success. Because of the intrusions attempting to nudge you from this zone, you will need to get adept at spending at least upwards of five minutes a day in the zone. The personal zone is not conferred by education because it is not earned in College, neither can it be conferred by any man. It is God-given and created in the mind.

FOCUS ON THE MOMENT

How do we focus without overly concentrating? And why do we think concentrating on this instance will defeat our mindfulness objective? It would produce more stress, which we are trying to reduce. Let's define the objective, and once defined, we will understand why concentration is counterproductive. We will identify the goals that will help us reach the objective. And by consistent practice, once or twice a day, this book will help you develop healthy mindfulness habits. When you focus on things outside yourself and the situations you find yourself in, or the people who form the circle of stress, you lose sight of your true objective. One's actual aim should be the healing peace that is to be found in the Oasis. Mind is the Oasis and the fountain that produces the raw diamonds we need as the investment for goal acquisition. Pragmatically focusing within, rather than without, brings a generic novelty to your opportunities and a freshness that your inner genius cherishes. It is the beginning of originality; but how do we control this? Without control, we would be playing and going nowhere. Control is a factor derived from what we may call the mindset. I intend to dedicate a whole chapter to the subject of mindset. One's attitude plays the role of a rudder for the mind as that instrument steers the boat on. So, we will cultivate the right mindset to obtain the best personal control we need to thrive. Why do we need control? We need control so we can stay within the circle of conscious endeavor. The circle of our immediate thought zone is the arena of focus If you study the picture carefully, you will notice the circular frame of the lens. This circular frame can represent 'boundaries' we can use to limit ourselves from straying from the 'zone'.

CONTROL

> **Stay within the Circle of conscious endeavor**

Why do we need control? We need control so we can stay within the circle of conscious endeavor. The circle of our immediate thought zone is the arena of focus If you study the picture carefully, you will notice the circular frame of the lens. This circular frame can represent 'boundaries' we can use to limit ourselves from straying from the 'zone'.

NO-ANXIETY ZONE

When we study our immediate environment, we understand how panic drives mania in Society today. Panic is a fear which originates in a lack of understanding or Not knowing. We saw how Ali Hafed jumped at the thought of searching the world for diamonds. It was a panicked decision but an ignorant one. There is an English adage that says:

"A bird in the hand is worth two in the bush"

It means to value what you have because it can provide you with more gains than the whims and dreams that sound so fantastic. Another way to put it is to use what you have to obtain what you need. Which is the one-line summary of Ali Hafed's story. Circumstances change when we step into purpose and stepping into purpose means knowing to lift a foot and follow it with the other foot once the first foot has landed. The key is to approach reality using **'One-Step-at-a-Time'**. The real focus is never desperate. It is never the product of desperate times. It is something that you willfully choose, and it is something that you choose consistently and continuously over an extended period. This consistency speaks of a skill acquired through practice and by little steps of repeated action. Developing a habit of a pensive pause when everything and everyone is in a rush is a demonstration of good critical thinking skills. I did a painting once and titled it 'Fishers'

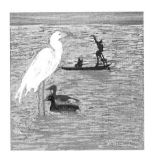

Fishers' by **WORDKRAFTER**

In that painting, you could see the three types of Fishers in the painting: The fishermen in the canoe, the Ducks searching for fish in the water, and the white Egret with eyes on distant fish below the waves in the river. If you can wrap your mind around the idea that you can choose to focus, you can start reclaiming the power you get when you focus by excluding distractions. Then we are not spending precious time worrying about things that may not happen since it does not bend time and make them happen. This is not a rewording of Murphy's Law! Simply put, it is a fact! Proactive worry is a negative application of the effectiveness of proactive preparedness. You do not have to sit around worrying about certain things that may or may not happen. By deciding, giving it the power attention deserves, and focusing the right number of resources and attention to detail, you end up getting the result you want without worrying yourself to death or having mental burnout. So, internalize your attention and calm the waters of each stressful moment, and you can focus your resources to the extent that you get much more results for your effort.

THE BOTTOM LINE

The bottom line with some focus is straightforward. You only have so many mental resources allocated to you within any given second; make them count! Learn whatever skills you need to get the most out of the time that you put into any activity. It is true that whatever attention you apply to any project or whatever resources you devote to your plans will pay off in solid returns. There is an economy of life that needs to be brought to bear by each individual on the way to life's success. But learning the skills one needs to succeed in those endeavors does not need to end in obtaining certification. One of the greatest tools for creating experts is called *ON-THE-JOB-LEARNING,* and Educationists call it *Learning-by-doing*. Many years ago while studying for my advanced Degree in Higher Education, I got familiar with the concept of Deep Learning. This occurs as a result of immersion into the material that needs to be learned. It occurs through cyclic iterative learning by doing the activity which is being learned.

APPLICATION: *YOU CAN SEE A CLEARER REALITY*

Observe the circle of your reality and endeavor to go beyond things that obscure your understanding. Endeavor to be conscious of your breathing. Seek understanding in each key moment, and you will establish key mileposts in the brain's wiring.

Our senses provide a fabric of synthesis for consciousness. While these senses enable each person to form his or her own reality, each one can learn to handle the brush strokes and color our reality wisely. As living beings we can add novel textures through *breath and emotion. These realities form our truth and lead us into our our grand designs. We are the architect of the design by using our inspirations to color the fabric or choosing not to. You can cultivate a different reality if you choose to.*

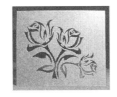

Chapter 6

THE HEALING MIND

As a Man thinketh, so he is

There are two perspectives on the healing mind. One is the perspective where the traumatized mind is continuously undergoing some form of repair, and the second one is where the mind confers healing, it's the instrument of healing. What these two perspectives are suggesting is that you can span trauma and the effects of trauma by your mindset. In the previous chapter, we spoke on the subject of cleansing, and as we give an opportunity to the mind cleansing itself, we allow inherent repair tools to provide a measure of healing. We always use the lens of focal objectivity to review our actions, dealing with them in the reality of the NOW ZONE, the ever-present moment of sensory perception. Unless we invest the right energy into our endeavors, we will continue to yield the wrong results. Being purpose-driven is a primary asset for success, but what is the purpose? The purpose is the reason for a mission, and it defines how and gives us a 'why' for doing the things we do. Unless the purpose is well identified from the beginning, there is a chance we may end up going nowhere. Think of it this way, when people show up at a funeral, and they see the deceased body in a box, what would you think people say about the Life he or she lived? Would you like them to say he/she was a kind person, or he /she helped a lot of people, or he/she revolutionized the World or discovered something? In the hearts of everyone is the truth. We need to think about these things while we are alive. This should form your grand objective because you are using other people's impressions of you as some sort of objective mirror for what you think you want for yourself.

MEMORY DETOX

Memories of the past should enable us to aim higher. When an Olympian Athlete looks at the records which were set in the past, he or she decides what the next goal should be. In our lives, we need to do a memory detox in which we accentuate the positives and eliminate the negatives. In other words, when you repeat your grand objective to yourself, think of memories as catalytic triggers. Zero in on one memory and ask yourself, " Did it happen?" Now, if the answer is 'yes', you need to analyze it further. But if the answer is 'no', then you need to start a process of de-cluttering and removing that which is best classified as 'fantasy'.This might be an assumed memory. You do not want to build a house on a foundation of loose sand. Now, assuming that the memory is based on facts and the things that did happen, ask yourself, 'What is the main lesson from this?' Every experience in Life is supposed to teach a lesson, so what is this teaching me?

ATTITUDE DETOX

Memory is one thing; attitude is another. Our attitude plays a big role in how Life turns out. If your attitude is that of a victim, then as Life turns out, you will find yourself feeling small, stuck, and powerless. Seek the bonus from every experience, for experience is more valuable than anything that money can buy. The hidden gems of Life are discovered when we visit the NOW ZONE daily. May your visits be rewarding and refreshing. These visits should be kept short and effective. My visits to the NOW ZONE are more effective when I use conscious breathing for at least 5 to 10 minutes.

WAYS OF THE HEALING MIND

The exquisiteness of the mind is that it bears within its recesses its own first-aid kit. You do not need a pill or any surgery to access this first-aid. It proceeds silently in those mysterious steps of thought. They are depicted as '**ways**' by me:

1. The first way of healing is *self-healing.*

Nature has blessed each one of us with a SELF-HEALING MIND. In order for the process of healing to proceed unhampered, the individual who needs healing has to *pull **out all the stops**.* These stops are the hindrances that get in the way of natural healing. What the mind needs is not bandaids, nor does it need clutter; clutter is anything that unnecessarily weighs the mind or distracts it from pristine functionality. The way nature has created our minds is unique for everyone and by free will, we can program our minds by learning through our portals of reality. These portals are the 5 senses: sight, smell, hearing, taste, and touch.

2. The second way is a ***mindset of healing***

Over the past 30 years, conscientious neurobiological research has shown that the placebo effect, a manifestation of an individual's mindset or expectation to heal, stimulates distinct brain areas associated with anxiety and pain that activate physiological effects that lead to healing outcomes. Mindsets can also lead to negative, or "nocebo," effects. For example, patients have been shown to have a heightened pain response after being informed that an injection will hurt. Those who were told about possible negative side effects of medication had an increased presence of those effects. The research continues to this day, with a lot of breakthroughs indicating that the mind possesses powers of healing based on self-programming or mindset.

3. The third way is the ***Learning mind***

The learning mind is the third way. The functional organ of the human mind is the brain, a thinking and living organism. Occupying the penthouse of the body, it is protected by a bony skull while stretching its wiring throughout the whole of the human body. Through the immense network of the mind's neurophysiology, the mind is a sentient organism. Through sensory nerves and through effector mechanisms, the brain applies its learning and is able to consciously apply healing effective processes. The mind is really an electromagnetic field that pervades the entire organism.

APPLICATION: *RESTORATION OF THE MIND*

The cluster of existence which is the mind is established as individual mindsets, and it is self-cleansing, self-healing, and self-learning. Above all it has consciousness. With Life comes a cloud of reality. Many names have been given to it, but none suffices. The attribute of Life confers many qualities to consciousness, and one thing is clear: Because we live, we have a mind and we must use the treasure trove of mental qualities to ensure a healthyy mindset.

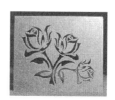

Chapter 7

MIND CLEANSING

Fresh beginnings n the Oasis

With the various anomalies which occur with excessive stress, we must stay vigilant and do all we can to help our minds stay sharp. One of the dulling pollutants is noise. According to Scientific America, noise affects brain activity, learning, memory and concentration levels. I struggled with the negative impact of noise after my stroke; suffering endless anguish even when the TV was not noisy to others. Even when two pople were engaged in loud conversation around me, I could not function. I have since then bought a series of ear muffs, noise canceling headphones and devised other methods so I can stay focused and productive. Not everyone will be as sensitive as I am to background noise, but most peple will be impacted, though they may not know it. My appeal is to you my dear reader. Even if you can surf the world and remain immune to the negative effects of noise, be an ambassador of quietness, As Max Erhmann says: *Go placidly....*

Mind cleansing is a term that means giving your brain a reboot from all clutter that is stressing you out, and hindering clearer thought. The feeling could come up suddenly and last a long time. Unless one tries to refresh the debris left behind by thoughts in the working memory, there will not be a clear field for fresh ideas. Just as a farmer has to plow his field and remove weeds or tree stumps before planting a new crop, one must be sure to clear the field of unwanted elements and create a fresh field. We sometimes want to clear our heads when looking for fresh ideas. It is the same thing. Fresh and viable ideation comes with fresh thoughts.

Earlier in the introduction, I mentioned that the human mind is a Quarterback. Like a Football Quarterback, the brain needs rest, refreshing, and revitalizing at intervals within the game. No athlete can play forever and not have breaks. We need to bring the practice of mindfulness into consonance with our Healing. In Chapter 5, we used the lens of focal objectivity to review our actions, dealing with them in the reality of the NOW zone. All the hard effort invested in each day's endeavor should yield more results than we see unless we invest the wrong type of energy. Being purpose-driven is a primary asset for success, but what is the purpose? The mind is intelligent; and unless it is well used, it will not serve its full purpose. Purpose creates the steps to meet the objectives of any mission, and it defines how, when, and if the mission is going to be accomplished. Purpose gives us a 'why' for doing the things we do. Unless the purpose is well identified from the beginning, we may go nowhere. In the previous chapter, you zeroed in on the grand objective of your Life and you zeroed in on what you want your life to produce. Think of it this way, when people show up at a funeral, and they see the deceased body in a box, what do you think people say about the Life he or she lived? Would you like them to say he/she was a kind person, or he /she helped many people, or he/she revolutionized the World or discovered something? In the hearts of everyone is the truth. We need to think about these things while we are alive. This should form your grand objective because you are using other people's impressions of you as some objective mirror for what you think you want for yourself.

MEMORY DETOX

Let us start with the inner recesses of mind. Memories of the past should enable us to aim higher. When an Olympian Athlete looks at the records which were set in the past, he or she decides what the next goal should be. In our lives, we need to do a memory detox to accentuate the positives and eliminate the negatives. In other words, when you repeat your grand objective to yourself, think of memories as catalytic triggers. Zero in on one memory and ask yourself, " Did it happen?" If the answer is 'yes,' you must analyze it further. But if the answer is 'no', then you need to start de-cluttering, removing that, which is best classified as fantasy. This might be an assumed memory. You do not want to build a house on a foundation of loose sand. Now, assuming that the memory is based on facts and the things did happen, ask yourself, 'What is the main lesson from this?' Every experience in Life is supposed to teach a lesson, so what is this teaching me?

ATTITUDE DETOX

The mirror that reflects the mind is our attitude. Memory is one thing; attitude is another because our attitude is the film that people watch all day long. Our attitude plays a big role in how Life turns out. If your attitude is that of a victim, then as Life turns out, you will feel small, stuck, and powerless. Seek the bonus from every experience, for experience is more valuable than anything money can buy. The hidden gems of Life are discovered when we visit the NOW ZONE daily, and the NOW ZONE is the ever-present moment in which all of life's happenings begin or end according to our perception. We will continue to explore the NOW ZONE paradigm and may all your visits be rewarding and as they are refreshing.

A CLEAN TOOL

A heling work of healing the human body proceeds under natural direction even if it is by medical or alternative means because only God heals. Take that to the bank! All caregivers and health Practitioners are stewards of Nature's propensity to heal and every tool from the medication, the scalpel to the procedures have to be clean. You my reader should employ a clean tool to! You may say *what is my tool?* I am glad you asked! There is a lot of research on the influence of the mind. One of such research areas is in the field of Epigenetics and Gene expression. Science has found that the way we think and behave has an effect on changes in our DNA and the way the body reads DNA. They have found that the way we grow old, fall sick and heal is due to theis genetic expression. I am including this in OASIS so as to inform you that your mind is a concrete tool in your wellness. Keep it clean by practicing a mindfulness that ensures proper gene expression. It will assist your longevity and healing.

APPLICATION: *CLEANER ATTITUDE AND SHARPER MEMORY*

Nurturing a clear mind and tending to your space allows you to think and act purposefully.

Give your mind a reboot by getting rid of the clutter of stress. The Quarterback has enough plays in his playbook. Enter the NOW ZONE.

A stream of water refreshes itself as it flows, and a stagnant body of water lasks freshness. By your mindful activities you will cause a flow of vitality that will make you more lively and productive. A cleaner attitude allows you to enhance your mindfulness therefore memory and recollection are improved. A clean mind is a tool of Wellness.

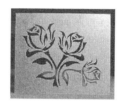

Chapter 8

MINDSET

Captain of Life's ship

William Ernest Henley was a 19th-century English poet, writer, critic, and editor. Though he wrote several books of poetry, Henley is remembered most often for his 1875 poem "Invictus". The last two lines contain invaluable advice to those who blame God for their failures. It is not only about God, but the mindset that makes us give up while faced with challenges. It is a proven fact that challenges make one stronger but mentally yielding oneself to those obstacles extinguishes the childlike enthusiasm that is the passionate inquisitiveness of all entrepreneurs. Through these lines, Henley shared that it's not about how difficult the path is, it's the momentum and attitude to keep moving forward without submitting oneself to fate's recourse. Attitude is synonymous with mindset. A mindset is a product of an "established set of attitudes". While taking some time to be established, mindsets eventually become habitual thus creating a cycle of mannerisms and behavioral patterns. These patterns eventually motivate or demotivate our choices.

When affliction strikes, the physical body could suffer to the extent that the conscious mind is unwilling to rise up to challenges. Sometimes this manifests as boredom, laziness of mind, or the lack of a will to fight an ailment. In my case in the early days of the stroke, I was depressed and anxious about what others would say. I am suggesting that one needs to prepare for that possibility. One needs a mindset, a practice that locks into the subconscious layers of protection. It is a proactive defense. If you are already afflicted and boredom is setting in, to the extent that you lack the will to survive; with the help of a Caregiver, encouragement should be provided to slowly get you into a survivor's mindset.

While attitude is synonymous with mindset, a mindset can be likened to the rudder of a ship. As we are the captains of our life's ships, the wise use of the rudder, in this case, the mind is of paramount importance. There is no perfect way to sail the ship of life, but you can have fun and learn while you are on the journey. Learn, learn, and learn! Use whatever knowledge you acquire for the benefit of mankind. You benefit mankind by being of service to others and caring for your environment. Speaking of our environment, each of our lives is a by-product of the environment we live in, Which is why the next section is a key addition to this book.

LIVING SPACES

One of the practices I would encourage you to adopt is tending to the spaces around you. As a tonic for the mind, we can borrow from some of the wisdom in Feng Shui the Japanese art of harmonizing our physical spaces. In Feng Shui, the Japanese people arrange the pieces in living spaces to create balance with the natural world. This is what it means to feng shui your home. The goal is to harness energy forces and establish harmony between individuals and their environment. They are not seeking aesthetics primarily. So we ask: what is the objective of the practice of Feng Shui? Why does an individual need to be in harmony with Nature?

SOME DETAILS ON FENG SHUI

Feng Shui is an ancient art that originated in China. It is over 6000 years old, and at its core are techniques and science of arranging objects and spaces in an environment to achieve optimal harmony and balance. In Chinese "Feng" means "wind" and "Shui" means "water." Its origins can be traced back to an ancient poem describing the feeling of being in harmony with nature. This philosophy is strongly influenced by Taoism. "Tao" means "the way" and Taoism refers to the "way of nature". The practice essentially creates harmony with nature in every living environment. For 6000 years Feng Shui rules guided the design of temples and ancient structures including the Great Wall of China. How does wisdom that built a 13,171-mile long wall still be effective after 3000 years in helping anyone who is reading OASIS right now?

APPLYING FENG SHUI

This book was written to bring together the 'meat' of applied mindfulness so anyone would be able to apply it as a pragmatic solution and a best practice for climbing out of the hole that sinks men and women in the vicious quicksands of modern-day hustle and bustle.

How can one apply the principles of Feng Shui to oneself in a winning strategy?

Feng Shui principles are based on practical methods which reflect on the mind's harmony.

RESTRUCTURING AND TRANSFORMING ONE'S ENVIRONMENT

By allowing the flow of energy from your environment to revitalize the mind. When you do this it will lead to the following:

- better sleep
- better mental health
- better productivity
- better overall health

START SMALL

Ask yourself the question: How does my living space look right now? Everyone should ask the same question periodically. It should be a never-ending inquiry that helps our continuous improvement mindset. This mindset does not assume perfection, does not procrastinate nor does it get frustrated. For the simple reason that it is a mindset that breaks obstacles into small manageable chunks. This helps identify specific and more accommodatable goals. Remember: Goals are the steps that you need to accomplish as you progress toward your vision. Allow me to branch out some supportive information. The reason for you to come to grips with the fundamental synergy that powers the mind is this: You are essentially your brain. This is why Rene Descartes, French philosopher, scientist, and mathematician pronounced his famous line in 1637: *Je pense, donc je suis*. Translated into the wider-read Latin of that time, it read: *Cogito, ergo sum*. This means **I think, therefore I am**.

Your thoughts are the fuel for your being, No wonder when we feel we are down in spirit, it is traceable to our thoughts, and in this book, we are exploring the connection between thoughts, mindfulness, and goal acquisition. Goal acquisition is the reward of our journey toward our vision. With mindset, we have a dual capability. The mindset acts as both the rudder and a compass. It is therefore important to adjust our mindsets regularly.

APPLICATION: *THE BEGINNING*

The environment of the mind is an arena of Conception , and it is where the birthing of purpose and healing takes place.

We all have a lot more in common than we think. Primarily we are all living things. With Life comes vitality and expression through our minds.

And because we all have a purpose for living, understanding brings a beginning of purposeful and productive steps.

Dreams, efforts and achievements can be birthed here or the could be destroyed. Dream big and feed your dreams. Speak to your vision with the language it understands. This is the language of your mindset. You should be the first person on the ship as well as the last man off it. You are the Captain of the ship which sets sail for your destiny.

Chapter 9

GOALS

Goals should lead to self-activating Objectives.

The use of objectives is commonplace in the world of business management, but it does not mean that laypeople cannot use goals effectively or manage their success with goals. We will not refer to their use in technical terms, but in simple and practical terms as it applies to success. Without this, each one of us may be the captain of life's ship, but then we would just sail through the waters of life and risk every storm without a plan. The whole mix of goals, objectives, and vision is simplified in OASIS. What everyone needs are self-activating objectives. You see, the management process of MBO (Management by objectives) is a process in which objectives trigger creativity with positivity and enthusiasm. The process takes a cue from the plan and gets activated to deliver the objective. There is a synergy of the elements within the plan. Almost as in perpetual motion, it keeps rising to the next level of success.

Would you not want to keep your focus on your vision, rising up each morning to a bright new day and full of hope for fulfilment and success. Through my belief and passion, I embody the precepts of effective management, trusting that any well-meaning individual can make use of this. I am including this chapter in this book because additionally, I found that it was my vision mix that kept me grounded as I healed from my illness. Blending positive energy with vision, objectives and goals is planning for success.

VISION

Before you launch out on the journey towards your most important venture, it is paramount that you describe your vision. No Ship Captain trusts his or her fate to the treacherous depth of any blue sea without having a reliable compass, enough fuel to get him to the next port, and a chart showing the route. In a nutshell, all this paraphernalia form the elements of a plan. We do not have to have the intention to sail the seven seas before we kit up the Ship. Proactivity with intention resolves to satisfaction in the end.You want to be able to measure your progress and identify helpful resources.

You need to celebrate your success and duplicate the process after learning to be effective and efficient.

These are basic factors that will help to draft the necessary plan. The plan starts by articulating your vision. A vision has to be described in explicit and descriptive terms which are to the planner's understanding. The clearer, the better and see your vision in your mind's eye as well. And since the mind's eye works best when the physical eye is shut, you have to visualize your plan in the previously referred to 'No Anxiety Zone'. This is a mental location between your conscious and subconscious mind. It is everywhere and nowhere. Let me explain; You can locate it wherever you are on the globe, but you need to be present. You see, the presence of the mind is a rare commodity nowadays. The reason is that anxiety kicks our presence of mind out of the window every time we seek a quiet moment. But OASIS is all about gaining the ability to sail a tranquil sea and the ability to find refuge away from turmoil.

BE LIKE WATER

The Japanese say Mizu No Kokoro. A phrase which means 'Be like the Water'. Water flows over every obstacle that forms a barrier in its path, or it wears it down over time. You should begin to practice this daily water mindfulness; in which you will slowly but surely become adept in the applications of the No-Anxiety-Zone. So, for the next three days, you must diligently practice the water mindfulness in your no anxiety zone.

MILEPOSTS

Spoken words are real; when people speak, sometimes those words resonate and sink into our being. These oftentimes upset us or may shatter our peace to the extent that the echo is transformed into a form of self-speak.

I do not know about you, but it could sometimes ruin my day to the extent that I am unable to fulfill some of my objectives.

I remember a prime example one morning when I had lined up a juicy to-do list. When I got in my car to head for the first milepost, starting what was intended to be a fulfilling day, I had to rethink. Though not an immediate rethink, all I could hear was the misleading, annoying, and false accusation from a close relative going out the door. The last thing I remembered was the accusation; everything else was a blur of fumbles after that. Even starting my car and coming out of the driveway at home, was a faint recollection; I even forgot my packed lunch, leaving it behind. After driving aimlessly having lost my to-do list in the endless maze of befuddled thoughts, I then decided to throw my plans for a fulfilled day out the window and return home to my oasis. I raise this little scenario to mention how people's words can affect our steps, our goals, and ultimately our Vision. We use the Chinese adage of a journey of a thousand steps and the fact that it begins with one step. The truth of it is made loud and clear, increments may accumulate slowly, and they are substantially important, but the wrong increments can lead to misdirection and loss of objective. In my case, on the morning in question I was getting a lot of misdirection from the wrong vibes. It was best to wipe the slate clean and start afresh. OASIS can help with that after you have read it and put the tips to practice. These are your daily steps or accomplishments toward your goals, Mileposts help to keep anyone who uses them, to keep on track to the next goal, and as goals are acquired, they will lead to the successful completion of our life missions. The joy and satisfaction begins before the completion. With each step and with each goal, like little rain drops, we gather water as our ship sails on to the final destination. A destination of fulfillment and satisfaction.

Here is a breakdown of the Vision paradigm for your use and understanding:

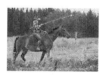

Your vision is like a carrot to a donkey. It provides the neccessary momentum and vitality the rider using the main the object in the donkey's view to excite the animal's passion achieve success in an essential endeavor. The carrot in this analogy is the best antidote for boredom, lack of interest and the bane of every worthy plan. First you should document the vision in writing. This is an aggreement with yourself. It is called a Charter.

CHARTER

Develop a charter, a document spelling out your vision concisely and include plan describing your mileposts vividly. So vividly that when you expect to reach them, they are very clear in your mind and when you pass them, they will be clear and vivid memorials for your encouragement. Personally, I recommend a piece of paper and a pen; there is a cognitive phenomenon known as the hand eye coordination. I have also tried the software approach, but whichever works best for you, go for it. When you creatively transcribe your vision into words or a picture or maybe a symbol, you are reflecting the language of the subconscious mind

APPLICATION: VITAL STEPS IN THE RIGHT DIRECTION

A journey of a thousand miles starts with one step. When we order and plan vital steps, the emergent picture depicts our vision with more clarity and measurement.

Little drops of water make up an ocean. Do not spend precious time on puny steps but spend mindful moments contemplating purpose and Vision and effectively planning vital steps.

Vital steps continuosly executed become a habit, and layers of healthy habits form a strengthen scaffold and a covering which empower men and women to live lives of activated energy and health.

There will be further fun-exercises for practicing goal setting based on the cocept of self activating objectives in the ***Oasis Workbook***.

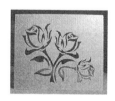

Chapter 10

CREATIVE VISUALIZATION

From a Bluepnt to Solid Realization

-

Everyone is an artist, painting a form of art which eventually become masterpieces for others to contemplate and for Almighty God to be proud of. Creativity is not a rare ability; it is what we are born to do. Living as creative beings, we are always creating things which were not there before. From the conversations we originate in our thoughts, as well as the words we speak, we are creators. These works of self-expression are unique to everyone.

What if I showed you something that can give you a shortcut to building creativity?

Why would you need to get more creative?

In the next few pages, we will find the information which will help form some answers to these questions.

All this is important because everyone is sitting on vast mind-potential energy which when developed needs to be deployed; and if not effectively deployed, will go to waste.

Would it not be nice if you could apply this newfound creativity in your job, your relationships, or your business?

I have come to understand that everyone has creativity on the inside, to some degree or another. We are all born with creativity, but many of us give it up because of endless reliance on our outer senses; what Psychologists term the objective mind. While in College, I was always fascinated by the projects of my Buddies in the Faculty of Architecture. These students were very creative, and while we in the Faculty of Pharmacy grabbed our Lab coats and set up for long experiments in Medicinal Chemistry or Pharmacognosy, those guys headed to their Design Rooms to build scaled models from their drawings. I had difficulty visualizing and translating their drawings into the 3-Dimensional models they painstakingly measured, cut, and glued. I struggled to link those 2-dimensional drawings to the fancy architectural models. They had it so well made that they had Palm trees, model lawns, and model cars sometimes in the garage. My Daughter, who is now an Architect, will guide me in this matter.

VISION BLUEPRINT

To aid this inherent creative propensity, we need to use effective visualization, and there is an art that will aid your creative visualization. With daily practice of this art form, you will attain greater proficiency, and over time you will truly be the

Captain of your ship. For over 50 years, I have been traveling this road, and I am getting better at converting my words, thoughts into visualized goals as Almighty God inspires me. I found out earlier on that there is a need to rehearse my objectives in small snapshots for them to become activated objectives. They are concretely activated as we breathe life into them! The steps which I am about to share with you will help in modeling the blueprint of each individual vision; I will list them as I have used them to sculpt my own vision from time to time.

Finally, visualizing your Vision daily allows you to hone the fine details, its precision, and the appeal to your passion; the lodestone steering your life's ship to destination. As I said earlier, your vision acts as the rudder of your life's ship. The more you visualize that vision, paying attention to the ephemeral details, the more the lodestone's effectiveness is established directing you to your final goal. And as the strokes of a magnet polarize a piece of iron to eventually become magnetic, repeated strokes of daily visualizing this Vision will cause you to be increasingly passionate and polarized. This increased polarization manifests as increased vitality, and you will start demonstrating increased energy and enthusiasm for your objective. The same phenomenon builds habits which have led successful people from the Marco Polo's of the World of Pioneering travel to the Leonardo DaVinci's of the World of Masterful Masterpieces. A mechanism which gets better by the day as we lay down each layer of visualization. In creative visualization, one should start each visualization as a draughtsman layer down each line with precision and finesse. Whether one is creatively working on the image of a red apple. It must eventually vibrate as a red apple in the mind's eye as the physical apple. The more practice with visualizing you get will one-day assistance by evoking the fragrance of a ripe apple.

FURTHER VISUALIZATION

I) Close your eyes and Imagine you are on a sandy beach at a lake on a sunny morning, the sky is clear, and though the Sun is shining, you can only feel a slight warmth on your face as the gentle breeze brings a slight fragrance to your nostrils.

In this exercise, you are not perceiving a physical scene but a mental scene. This is why you had to close your eyes and use creative visualization. Whenever you repeat this exercise, you may include other details of your choice in the picture. The important thing is that you should try to repeat the same details going forward.

When you have succeeded in achieving good visualization, you are ready to apply this technique to manifest your life's vision. This exercise is dynamic as well as cumulative. You should start by creating a picture in your mind representing the simplest idea of your Vision.

II) Also, whenever you have an idle moment, maybe you are having to kill time in a Doctor's waiting room, and it is taking forever to be attended to, then you can apply the second strategy for your creative visualization. I suggest you use the help of a piece of blank paper and a pen. I want you to create a symbol that best represents your vision of what you want. Keep it as simple as possible, it is only a symbol. Try to complete your symbol in the little time before it gets to be your turn in the queue. After you are satisfied with the symbol and you are convinced it represents your vision, keep going over every aspect of the diagram, then tuck it away in your pocket. Do not lose it but seize the opportunity to review your vision symbol over the next few days. The more it agrees with you, the more it will resonate in your subconscious.

That is when it simulates a beacon for your life's ship, just as lighthouses beckoned and guided sail ships in the early years. I will discuss how this simple operation can be used as an aid to draw you closer to your vision later on. I call this exercise **VISION DOODLE**. If you think you may not be able to doodle, you can clip a photo from a magazine that depicts your vision. As an example, here is my own Vision Doodle as I aspire to be an Author.

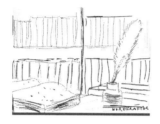

APPLICATION: VISON DOODLE

The mind thinks in pictures. You need to have a creative trigger that stimulates your mind's eye. The effect will enhance your appetite for success. The Vision Doodle will spur you to better achieve your goals.

Through Creative visualization in as little as ten days, you will be able to create the masterpiece of your vision. The joy of accomplishing your life purpose should be realized even while you are on the journey to your destination. The added joy at every milepost, as you approach, the vision grants you an extra stimulus. Practice Creative Visualization daily to get proficient at it!

Everyone is an artist, painting a masterpiece for others to contemplate and for Almighty God to be proud of. Creativity is not a rare ability, it is what we are born to do. In this creative being, we are creating something that was not there before. From the conversations we originate from our thoughts and the words we speak, we are creators. These works of self-expression are unique to everyone.

What if I showed you something that has been helping me build extra strength in creativity for more than fifty years, granting you a few shortcuts to creative expression?

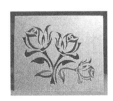

Chapter II

CARING

It takes two

I have been writing the script for this book for some time now and then I thought I should cap my efforts with a very important chapter. This topic is really what makes the difference between a superficial attempt at healing, prevention, or thriving and why so many fail. We are the best caregivers of ourselves, in the first place. Any caregiver taking care of a patient or stroke survivor will depend on this critical element. No one can read another's mind, pain, or suffering as precisely as the individual going through it. Therefore;

every attempt at caring should encourage openness, trust, and dependability.

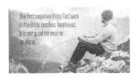

At one time or the other, most families have to care for one other family member. God has ordained family, and the Holy Bible lets us know this in the Book of Beginnings when He said: "It is not good for Man to be alone" [Genesis 2: 18]. This statement was not just alluding to a wife but was a creative and prophetic masterpiece by the Creator of all, directed at the wellbeing of the total man, and spoken in the time of the beginning of all beginnings. Caring, especially when it is done with the utmost compassion, goes a long way to healing the wounds of life and the mind.

I wish to address a subunit of caring and one which is most pertinent to the basic plan of the natural ecology of man. I say natural ecology as meaning not man-made. The natural ecology is made up of the internal and external aspects of the physiology of man, and since OASIS was born out of inspiration Germain to the throes of the affliction known as a stroke, I will bring the caring theme home.

My experience initially brought on a heavy cloud of depression. The very things I counseled my mentees on had now afflicted me in the heaviest of ways. From the integrative wellness side was the sucker punch of the depressing notion that I was now a virtual hypochondriac prescribed a daisy chain of medications. Each pill was an attempt to swat the virtual flies which swirled around my physiology. I had been a staunch disciple of a medicinal plant regimen having specialized in medicinal plants in my Pharmacy degree. With the daisy chain of prescriptions, my challenge was having to remember to take every medication on time and in the proper sequence. With my Aphasia, I had the tendency to have a brain fog in which I lost track of time or the things I had done.

I bring this out in OASIS because one of the things I realized in the early days of survival was that my recovery was not just based on my medications but on a sequence of what I termed Vital Recovery Steps [VRS].

VRS
Vital Recovery Steps

What are vital recovery steps? They are steps leading to recovery, which synergistically make a tremendous difference, larger than if they were not taken at all. They end up propelling our natural wellness and aid the accomplishment of the positive outcomes we expect. The same principle can be used for any affliction because it is simply leveraging Nature's resourcefulness and masterful design. You see as I often tell my Stroke Support group, Nature is a Masterful Watchmaker. In Man, the design has an in-built proactive repair which rises up to adverse states, rectifying anomalies, and deficiencies,

One concept which helped me in my stroke recovery was Neurogenetic Neuroplasticity. Under this understanding, I developed a mindset to leverage the brain's ability to regenerate and build new nerve strands based on mind science. As an example, I will enumerate my own vital steps later because these steps are vital to my recovery. For you, you may need to assemble your own bio-individual steps. To everyone a different set of vital steps. I cite my own vital steps just to let you know I applied a consistent science and so should you.

VRS: strategies to help self-recovery or for others to recover from physical, mental nd emotional disabilities. One can use creative visualization exercises to help focus on one's own Vision daily, while rehearsing the vital steps and previous achievements and at every opportunity. Then, we should collect available tools to design some innovative ways to overcome gaps in effectiveness.

My tools for example, were: text-to-speech software, color writing pens, noise canceling earplugs, and a collection of Bonsai for a hobby. Even after survival of an adverse medical condition, and recovery starts , one will need to plan for prevention while following Doctors' advice and prescriptions as precisely as possible. So, aids that help memory such as diaries, alarm clocks and color-codes certainly help.

Designing your own vital recovery steps will help you to stretch those cognitive boundaries which limit wellbeing and attempt to surmount limitations daily

Every opportunity should be adopted to communicate with known and unknown people regularly. Speech is golden.

COMPASSION

When caregivers show compassion, they help the healing process. I had many people help with my healing, but healing starts at home and with family. My wife Anella helps me daily surmount the rigors of survival.

APPLICATION: Recovery is a step-at-a-time

What is a mentally visualized Vision? A mentally visualized vision as opposed to a vision written on paper is a vision that exists only in the mind. When it is in the mind and not on paper, it activates the mind better and faster than the one on paper.

A well-rehearsed vision is one in which its owner can mentally call it up wherever he or she is.

With the help of innovative ways, handicaps may be overcome easier while constantly stretching and challenging the cognitive boundaries to one's abilities.

Do not forget to work the communication tool, for family, neighbors and society at large forms a healing network. Every Caregiver must always encourage the handicapped person being cared for, to keep the vision of hope alive. Remember; the little steps matter the most.

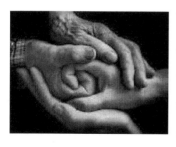

When caregivers show compassion, they help the healing process. I had many people help with my healing, but healing starts at home and with family. My wife Anella helps me daily surmount the rigors of survival.

APPLICATION: Recovery is a step-at-a-time

1. What is a mentally visualized Vision? A mentally visualized vision as opposed to a vision written on paper is a vision that exists only as the mind. When it is in the mind and not on paper, it lives as opposed to the one on paper.

2. A well-rehearsed vision is one in which its owner can mentally call it up wherever he or she is.

3. With the help of innovative ways, handicaps may be overcome

4. Constantly stretching and challenging cognitive boundaries will improve one's abilities

5. When one communicates with known

and unknown a network opens

A Caregiver must always encourage the handicapped person being cared for, so as to keep the vision of hope alive. Remember; the little steps matter the most, because they add up and are vital opportunities for continuous improvement.

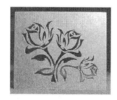

Chapter 12

TOOLS

Keeping the Mind in shape

Keeping in shape is not only important if someone intends to turn into a circus wonder or get conferred with a body-building World title. Right under our noses is the wonder of wonders, if only we can tend to its fitness. This wonder of wonders sits in a box which is able to withstand over 500 pounds of pressure.

The Human Brain is the wonder of wonders and an American poet Emily Dickinson, in a poem written around 1892, described the wonder of the human brain.

Emily was a reclusive poet. Only a recluse would lack the distraction of societal living enough to recognize the beauty and strength which is mankind's blessing. Anyone reading these verses should know they share in a miraculous work of Creation. Everyone should treat his or her Brain as such. We marvel at some of the things this organism can accomplish, and we can only realize the tip of the iceberg. It is a colossus of creativity and the snowflake of ingenuity, capable of unimaginable but astounding configuration in its manifold extensions. Musing on how this fascinating organ is able to encompass so much information about the self and the world, she wrote:

> "The Brain -is wider than the sky
>
> For- put them side by side-
>
> The one the other will contain
>
> With ease- and you- beside."

Emily Dickinson

HARDWARE/SOFTWARE

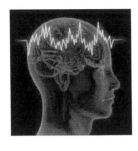

Nature plants seeds in Creation for germination and fruition. So also, does she plant seeds in our consciousness for inspiration and germination. The knowledgeable man uses the seeds planted in his consciousness for food, the wise man uses the same thing to form a life but the man or woman who would be great uses it to build himself or herself and society at large. The seed of OASIS has grown into a conceptual tree, the fruit of which are these notions:

The grey matter of the Brain is the hardware

The mind is the software, and it flows with consciousness

UPDATE / UPGRADE

Everything about you tells a subtle story. Your name is not written on your forehead, yet when you look at your face in the mirror, the subtle characteristics of your face speak loud and clear. You recognize who you are and not someone else. But there is more to it than meets the eye here, for every experience that wafted its way through to the hidden screen of your mind has carved invisible records and etched definite lines into your brain by way of the subconscious mind. These lines form a definite trait map of who you really are. That is why the hardware of the Brain should regularly be updated. How do you upgrade the hardware of the Brain?

Certainly not by attaching other hardware, but by supplementation and nutrition. Nutritive sources provide specific molecules that energize and tone the Brain. We do not have the space or the time to do an extensive package here about the subject, but I will give some tips on how to keep the brain ticking in its prime. After this, we will address the subject of updating the Brain.

Upgrading the Brain boosts cognitive power by increasing the level of acetylcholine the communication enzyme which powers it.

Nature plants seeds in Creation for germination and fruition. So also does she plant seeds in our consciousness for inspiration and germination. The knowledgeable man uses the seeds planted in his consciousness for food, the wise man uses the same thing to form a life but the man or woman who would be great uses it to build himself or herself and society at large. The seed of OASIS has grown into a conceptual tree, the fruit of which are these notions:

The grey matter of the Brain is the hardware

The mind is the software, and it flows with consciousness

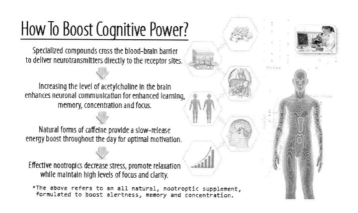

Updates to the brain help improve what the brain knows. This is achieved by feeding it with facts and data. Together upgrades and updates create a healthier Brain. There are also apps such as Luminosity which provide exercises for brain health. Brainhq is another one and has free exercises online.

CHANGERS YOU CAN MAKE TO YOUR BRAIN	
UPDATE THE BRAIN	Feed it information and by exercise
UPGRADE THE BRAIN	Nutrition & Supplementation

In order for the Brain to function smoothly, we must have Brain updates as well as Brain upgrades.

To assist in this-wise you should download the OASIS Workbook, which is available online at :

Https://www.TEMGUN.com

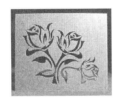

Chapter 13

FINAL WORDS

You can do it

The steps in OASIS are simple, but they are not easy. Diamonds are created from carbon by a Creator who hides His simplicity in complexity and from the same elements in charcoal. To some of my readers, the skill of finding keywords will be easy and almost magical. to others, it could mean a lot of hours of note-taking and practice. Believe me, it was the same for me. This is a tried and tested road and a road that works. you will find refreshing in tiresome stressful moments through the pages of OASIS. All the stress and pain which lead to my truth are not replicated in this book, but their revelation is distilled for anyone who will take some time to read it.

With these final words, it is now your turn to be a Doer. It has been a rigorous time writing sleeping on my thoughts on paper, collating research, and validating my experience. I have journeyed through the pages of this book, traveling through the desert sands of time and trying to tell it as it is. This has not been teaching but an account of my actual steps. Rather than sweating through a desert experience, I have pointed you in the direction of an OASIS near you.

I had to do this final chapter because I how much I believe in you. Whatever your reason for venturing into the Oasis of the mind, let me assure you: you can do it. Every Olympic athlete has a vision that is so dynamic that they always face daunting odds right from the start. The vision is so dynamic that no sooner than they have set an outstanding record than they are looking at the next milepost 0f improvement. This is an attribute I want you to adopt. And as you adopt this attribute you are going to make continuous improvement the cornerstone of your excellence.

As a final recap let us piece together key points from all the chapters. It will serve as a type of Synopsis.

SYNOPSIS: *All we have discussed*

- **INTRODUCTION**: The concept of a **QUARTERBACK**- The Brain has a playbook in the recesses of memory. Also, the thought was developed about showing that mindfulness helps the brain to create significant mileposts on life's journey to our vision.

1. **DUALITY OF MIND**: Observing the Sunrise as an exercise of **Mindfulness**.

2. **THE PRECIOUS MIND:** Goals are **MILEPOSTS** that tell us how we are doing on the way to our vision.

3. **THE FOCUSED MIND:** Focus helps

us to stay within the **CIRCLE OF CONSCIOUS ENDEAVOR**

4. **MIND CLEANSING:** Give your Brain a fresh **REBOOT**.

5. **THE HEALING MIND**: **PURPOSE** always aims higher.

6. **MINDSET:** You are the Captain of the ship of your life and your rudder is your **MINDSET.**

7. **GOALS:** Be like **Water.**

8. **CREATIVE VISUALIZATION:** Visualize your Vision Daily.

9. **CARING:**

With this synopsis, I wish you a refreshing time as you journey through life and across the dry spots. May you find an oasis to refresh your efforts along the way and as you prepare for your next journey.

Though the writing of this script is almost over, it is only the beginning of new things for you and I am excited for you because I know that if Nature has fashioned your mind so beautifully, the best is yet to come as potential unfolds in its exquisite beauty. The concept of OASIS is entirely based on an inbuilt ability of the human mind for regeneration and renewal. The mind does this by utilizing internal natural resources known to Science as neurogenesis in a phenomenon known as neuroplasticity demonstrated by the Brain.

As I said earlier, I am not a neuroscientist but I have learned to stand on the shoulders of giants and learn as I follow the path they have trod. So as I travel life's path, I point the way ahead to you. The way ahead is a way of peace and a way that will allow each one of my readers to flourish, as potential dictates.

You are the captain of your ship. Indeed you set your course by your vision, aspiring and affirming by the dictates of potential as you journey each step and each goal of life. No one can stop you except you surrender by choice. You were built to excel, therefore do not stunt your growth. An Acorn was not meant to remain a seed, but a mighty Oak.

Thank you for patiently reading this book, and I look forward to the success stories which I know will surely come, as surely as there is an Oasis in every desert. You are not a mirage; You are real, and I wish you all the best in your achievements.

APPLICATION: A refreshing; a-day-at-a-time

The journey of life is a day-to-day and a step-by-step venture. As the Captain of your life ship, use the 8 synoptic applications above to journey from Oasis to Oasis while finding refreshment from time to time. May your refreshing be inspirational and revitalizing.

Thank you for taking time to read OASIS. The book is a practical summary of how to find refreshening in difficult times. In order to acquire the OASIS Mindset, and a mindset that is refreshing itself daily, please make it a worthwhile objective to obtain the OASIS WORKBOOK. This is a concise tool for practicalizing the tools you were introduced to within OASIS. As you practice with these tools you will be established in your new lifestyle. A lifestyle which prevents stress and sustains wellness. May you be refreshed indeed.

[The Author]

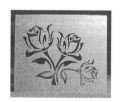

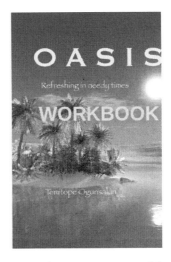

Request the OASIS Workbook

Https://www.TEMGUN.com/workbook

or

Email: bak2newwellness @me.com

Chapter 15

RESOURCES

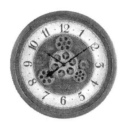

The image of a clock has been used to represent all the resources pertaining to OASIS because time itself is a resource which is vital to the affairs of mankind. Below is a list of some of the references that have been used as part of my research for OASIS.

American Heart Association https://youtu.be/AcbsUHOajW8

Balzer, D. (2022, March 30). Expert discuses Aphasia. Aphasia. Retrieved April 15, 2023, from: https://newsnetwork.mayoclinic.org/discussion/a-mayo-clinic-expert-explains-aphasia/

CDC Stroke facts https://www.cdc.gov/stroke/facts.htm

Chopra, D., & Tanzi, R. E. (2013). Super brain. Sperling & Kupfer.

Dananjaya, W. M. S., & Veerasingam, E. B. The Projection of Subconscious through Symbolism: An Analysis of Mansfield's 'The Voyage.'. International Journal of Scientific and Research Publications (IJSRP), 8(11).

Kabat-Zinn, J. (2009). Wherever you go, there you are Mindfulness meditation in everyday life. Hachette UK.

Leaf, C. (2013). Switch on your brain: The key to peak happiness, thinking, and health. Baker Books.

Paulson, S., Davidson, R., Jha, A., & Kabat-Zinn, J. (2013). Becoming conscious: the science of mindfulness. Annals of the New York Academy of Sciences, 1303(1), 87-104.

Syn-O-Vate (2021) Bringing together the jigsaw of life: Blog by Dr. T. Ogunsakin [Temgun.com: https://www.temgun.com]

Walters, A. S. (2021). The inner sounds of silence. The Brown University Child and Adolescent Behavior Letter, 37(11), 8-8.

Made in the USA
Columbia, SC
02 February 2024